SOUND THERAPY

A Comprehensive Guide to Sound Therapy -
Unveiling Ancient Wisdom, Modern Science,
and Practical Techniques for Healing,
Relaxation, and Transformation

WILFREDO CARSON

The book "Sound Therapy with Expert Guidance" delves deeply into the essence of sound healing, examining its history, efficacy, and profound benefits. Through a comprehensive lens, readers are introduced to the fundamental principles of sound, from the physics behind it to its pivotal role in centuries-long cultural practices.

This enlightening journey centers on the tools and instruments of sound therapy, which are meticulously dissected to reveal their unique vibrational properties and healing potential. From the ethereal resonance of singing bowls to the rhythmic cadence of drums, readers are empowered to explore and select instruments that resonate with their individual needs. Practical guidance on maintenance and care ensures that these instruments become enduring companions on the pa

The book delves into the realm of techniques and practices, offering a rich tapestry of sound-based modalities for personal and professional growth. From the sublime experience of sound bathing to the precise science of binaural beats, readers are equipped with a diverse toolkit to navigate the complexities of modern life with grace and resilience.

In this book, readers are invited to embark on a journey of self-discovery and renewal, from cultivating a healing environment to harnessing the therapeutic power of sound in meditation and yoga. Integrating sound therapy into daily life is a cornerstone of this transformative journey, where sacred rituals and healing practices converge to create a sanctuary of inner peace.

The book serves as a beacon of hope for stress relief and anxiety management.

Sound therapy's profound impact on physical, emotional, and neurological well-being is central to the narrative, offering solace to those grappling with chronic illnesses and mental health challenges. Through poignant case studies and success stories, the transformative potential of sound therapy is vividly brought to life, offering a ray of hope to those seeking healing and wholeness. Ethical considerations and professional standards highlight the importance.

In essence, "Sound Therapy with Expert Guidance" is more than just a book—it is a beacon of light in a world shrouded in darkness, offering a path to healing, transformation, and transcendence. Through its pages, readers are invited to embark on a journey of self-discovery and empowerment, guided by the timeless wisdom of sound and the compassionate expertise of seasoned practitioners. As the harmonious melodies of healing resonate through the soul, may we find solace.

Introduction

Sound Therapy is a multifaceted discipline that integrates ancient wisdom, modern science, and practical techniques to facilitate healing, relaxation, and transformation. With roots deeply embedded in various cultures and traditions across the globe, sound has long been recognized for its profound effects on the human psyche and physiology.

This comprehensive guide aims to explore the complexities of Sound Therapy, shedding light on its historical significance, therapeutic

Understanding Sound Therapy

At its core, Sound Therapy encompasses a diverse range of approaches that use sound vibrations to induce therapeutic effects on the mind, body, and spirit, including techniques such as chanting, singing bowls, tuning forks, and sound baths, among others.

The fundamental principle underlying Sound Therapy is the notion that sound is a vibrational phenomenon capable of influencing the energetic balance within the human system, rather than just an auditory experience.

What Is Sound Therapy?

Sound Therapy is the intentional use of sound frequencies to stimulate physiological and psychological responses that promote healing and well-being. Unlike traditional forms of medicine, which often target specific symptoms or ailments, sound therapy takes a holistic approach that addresses the individual as a whole, acknowledging the interconnectedness of mind, body, and spirit.

The History And Evolution Of Sound Healing

The history of sound healing can be traced back to ancient civilizations, where sound was revered for its sacred and therapeutic properties. Indigenous cultures all over the world incorporated chanting, drumming, and vocal toning into their rituals and ceremonies, recognizing the profound impact these practices had on consciousness and well-being. Over time, various spiritual traditions and healing modalities emerged, each offering unique perspectives on the power of sound.

Benefits And Effectiveness Of Sound Therapy:

Sound therapy has a wide range of advantages, including the ability to induce altered states of consciousness and reduce stress, lower blood pressure, and promote relaxation by activating the body's natural relaxation response. It can also aid in the release of stored tension and trauma, resulting in greater emotional resilience and well-being.

How Does Sound Therapy Work?

Sound Therapy's mechanisms are multifaceted and complex, involving both physiological and energetic processes. At a physiological level, sound waves interact with the body's tissues and organs, producing measurable effects on heart rate, brainwave activity, and hormonal balance. Entrainment, where external rhythms synchronize with internal rhythms, can help restore coherence and harmony within the body-mind system.

Overview Of The Book:

In this comprehensive guide to sound therapy, readers will embark on a journey of exploration and discovery, delving into the rich tapestry of sound healing practices from around the world.

From ancient wisdom traditions to cutting-edge scientific research, each chapter offers valuable insights and practical techniques for harnessing the transformative power of sound.

CHAPTER 1
THE FUNDAMENTALS OF SOUND

Understanding the fundamentals of sound, which is a mechanical wave that propagates through a medium like air, water, or solids, is essential for understanding its therapeutic applications. Sound is a fundamental aspect of human perception and communication, serving as a crucial element in various aspects of life, from language to entertainment and, most importantly, therapy.

<u>The Physics Of Sound:</u>

The physics of sound is the study of the intricate mechanisms by which sound waves propagate and interact with their surroundings. Sound waves have several key properties: frequency, which is the number of oscillations or cycles of a wave per unit of time and is typically measured in Hertz (Hz), amplitude, which is the magnitude or intensity of a sound wave and determines its perceived loudness, and wavelength, which is the spatial distance between success

<u>Properties of sound waves:</u>

Sound waves have distinct characteristics that affect their perception and effects on the human body and mind. Frequency determines the pitch of sound, with higher frequencies corresponding to higher pitches and vice versa; amplitude governs the loudness or intensity of sound, influencing its impact on the listener; and wavelength, while less directly perceptible, contributes to the tonal quality and timbre of sound. These properties interact dynamically to shape the audit.

<u>Understanding resonance:</u>

In sound therapy, resonance is used to elicit physiological and psychological responses in individuals by matching the frequency of the external force with the natural frequency of the object, resulting in amplified vibrations.

<u>The Function of Sound in Healing:</u>

Throughout history, sound has been revered for its healing properties, and diverse cultures have incorporated sonic rituals into their traditional healing practices.

From chanting and drumming to the use of instruments such as singing bowls and tuning forks, sound therapy encompasses a rich tapestry of techniques aimed at promoting physical, emotional, and spiritual wellness.

Ancient civilizations believed in the innate power of sound to restore harmony and balance within

Ancient Practices and Cultural Beliefs:

From the rhythmic drumming of African tribes to the chanting of Vedic mantras in India, sound therapy has its roots in the annals of human history, tracing back to ancient civilizations across the globe.

The Egyptians, Greeks, and Indigenous peoples of the Americas all used sound in rituals and ceremonies, recognizing its profound influence on consciousness and healing.

Modern Scientific Validation:

In recent decades, advances in scientific research have shed light on the efficacy and mechanisms underlying sound therapy.

Neuroscientific studies have elucidated the neural correlates of auditory perception and processing, revealing the profound impact of sound on brain function and behavior.

Clinical trials have demonstrated the therapeutic benefits of sound therapy in diverse populations, ranging from individuals with chronic pain and anxiety disorders to those

CHAPTER 2
SOUND THERAPY TOOLS AND INSTRUMENTS

Sound therapy, also known as sound healing or sound meditation, is a holistic healing practice that utilizes various sound tools and instruments to promote relaxation, alleviate stress, and facilitate physical, emotional, and spiritual well-being. The instruments used in the process are central to the effectiveness of sound therapy, as each offers unique vibrations and frequencies that interact with the human body on a profound level.

This section will delve into the various

From ancient civilizations to modern wellness practices, the use of sound as a healing modality has persisted and evolved. Sound therapy instruments are a diverse range of tools designed to produce harmonious sounds and vibrations conducive to healing and relaxation. They have been used for centuries across various cultures and traditions, reflecting the universal recognition of sound's therapeutic potential.

Singing bowls, originating from Tibetan and Himalayan cultures, are among the most recognizable and widely used sound therapy instruments. When struck or rubbed with a mallet, these bowls emit resonant tones, which are believed to synchronize brain waves, induce meditative states, and harmonize the body's energy centers or chakras. Practitioners frequently incorporate sing

Tuning forks are precision-crafted metal instruments with two prongs that vibrate at specific frequencies when struck against a surface. These frequencies are based on mathematical calculations and correspond to musical notes or therapeutic tones. In sound therapy, tuning forks are used to stimulate acupressure points, balance the body's energy flow, and facilitate deep relaxation.

The application of tuning forks can range from direct placement on

Drums and percussion instruments have a long history of use in ceremonial rituals, spiritual practices, and healing ceremonies worldwide. The rhythmic patterns and vibrations generated by drums can entrain brainwave activity, induce trance states, and promote emotional release. In sound therapy, drums and percussion instruments are used to ground, energise, and facilitate cathartic experiences.

Whether through shamanic drumming, frame drumming,

Gong baths, immersive experiences in which participants lie surrounded by the reverberating sounds of gongs, have grown in popularity in modern sound therapy settings. Gongs are revered in Asian cultures for their auspicious symbolism and therapeutic properties. The deep, resonant tones produced by gongs are thought to penetrate the body at a cellular level, promoting relaxation, releasing tension, and restoring balance.

Chimes and bells, with their delicate yet penetrating sounds, are cherished for their ability to uplift the spirit and clear stagnant energy.

Used in various spiritual and meditative traditions, these instruments produce pure tones that soothe the mind and uplift the spirit. In sound therapy, chimes and bells are employed for their purifying and harmonizing effects, which promote mental clarity and enhance the overall sense of well-being.

Choosing the Right Instruments: Choosing the appropriate sound therapy instruments requires careful consideration of various factors, including the practitioner's intention, the client's needs, and the desired therapeutic outcomes. Each instrument carries its own unique qualities and vibrational properties, which may resonate differently with individuals based on their preferences and sensitivities. Practitioners often choose instruments

Considerations to Consider: Practitioners may assess the suitability of sound therapy instruments based on factors such as the client's preferences and sensitivities, the therapeutic goals of the session, and the specific techniques employed. For instance, individuals with a strong affinity for melodic sounds may respond well to singing bowls or chimes, while those seeking deep relaxation may benefit from the grounding effects of drums or gongs. Additionally,

Depending on the instrument's material and construction, maintenance tasks may include polishing metal surfaces, replacing worn mallets or strikers, and storing the instrument in a dry, temperature-controlled environment.

In conclusion, sound therapy instruments are powerful tools for promoting healing, relaxation, and transformation.

Whether through the soothing tones of singing bowls, the rhythmic vibrations of drums, or the celestial sounds of gongs and chimes, these instruments offer diverse avenues for accessing the profound effects of sound on the body, mind, and spirit. By understanding the origins, mechanisms, and therapeutic applications of sound therapy instruments, practitioners can

CHAPTER 3
TECHNIQUES AND PRACTICE
Basic Sound Therapy Techniques

Sound therapy encompasses various techniques aimed at utilizing sound vibrations to promote healing, relaxation, and overall well-being. One fundamental practice is sound bathing, where individuals immerse themselves in a sonic environment created by various instruments such as singing bowls, gongs, or tuning forks. This immersive experience allows the body and mind to synchronize with the frequencies produced, inducing a state of deep relaxation and mental clarity. Vocal toning, another basic technique, involves the intentional production of sustained vocal sounds to resonate with specific areas of the body, thereby facilitating energetic balance and release of tension. Mantra chanting, derived from ancient spiritual traditions, involves the repetition of sacred sounds or phrases, which are believed to have profound transformative effects on the psyche and spirit. Guided meditation with sound combines traditional meditation practices with the use of soundscapes or music designed to evoke specific emotional states or promote inner peace. These basic sound therapy techniques form the foundation of sound healing practices, offering accessible avenues for individuals to explore the therapeutic potential of sound vibrations.

Advanced Techniques.

In addition to basic sound therapy techniques, advanced practices leverage cutting-edge technology and scientific understanding to further enhance the therapeutic benefits of sound. Binaural beats, a prominent advanced technique, involve the presentation of two slightly different frequencies to each ear, resulting in the perception of a third frequency known as the binaural beat. This phenomenon has been shown to entrain brainwave patterns, potentially leading to states of relaxation, focus, or heightened creativity. Brainwave entrainment, closely related to binaural beats, encompasses various methods of synchronizing brainwave activity with external stimuli, such as sound pulses or light flashes. By aligning brainwave frequencies with desired mental states, such as alpha for relaxation or gamma for heightened cognition, this technique offers a powerful tool for optimizing cognitive function and emotional well-being. Sound frequency therapy, another advanced approach, involves the precise application of specific frequencies to target physiological or psychological imbalances within the body. Drawing on principles from physics and bio resonance, practitioners utilize frequency generators or specialized instruments to deliver therapeutic frequencies, potentially facilitating cellular repair, stress reduction, or emotional release.

These advanced techniques exemplify the intersection of ancient wisdom and modern science in the realm of sound therapy, offering innovative solutions for addressing a wide range of health and wellness concerns.

Sound therapy encompasses a diverse array of techniques, ranging from basic practices rooted in ancient traditions to advanced methods informed by contemporary research and technology.

Whether through immersive soundscapes, vocal toning, or brainwave entrainment, the therapeutic potential of sound vibrations continues to inspire exploration and innovation in the fields of health and wellness. Understanding and harnessing the power of sound, individuals can

CHAPTER 4
INTEGRATING SOUND THERAPY INTO EVERYDAY LIFE

Integrating sound therapy into daily life entails incorporating various sound-based practices and techniques into one's routine to promote overall well-being. This concept revolves around the idea that sound, whether through music, chanting, or specific frequencies, can have profound effects on the mind, body, and spirit.

<u>Creating sacred space:</u>

Creating a sacred space for sound therapy entails setting up an environment that is conducive to relaxation, healing, and spiritual connection. This space can be physical, such as a dedicated room or corner of a room, or it can be created mentally through intention and mindfulness. The key is to cultivate an atmosphere that feels safe, serene, and supportive, allowing individuals to fully immerse themselves in the healing power of sound.

<u>Setting Up a Healing Environment:</u>

Setting up a healing environment for sound therapy entails creating conditions that facilitate relaxation, rejuvenation, and inner balance. This includes both the physical space in which sound therapy takes place and the atmosphere that is cultivated within it. Lighting, temperature, and sound quality can all contribute to the overall effectiveness of the healing environment. Additionally, incorporating elements such as natural materials, soothing colors

<u>Using Sound in Meditation and Yoga Practice:</u>

Sound has been used for centuries as a powerful tool for meditation and yoga, helping to deepen relaxation, promote concentration, and facilitate spiritual growth. It can take various forms, such as chanting mantras, listening to ambient music, or using specific sound frequencies to entrain brainwaves. By incorporating

<u>Sound Therapy for Stress Reduction:</u>

Sound therapy for stress relief involves using sound-based techniques to alleviate the physical, emotional, and mental symptoms of stress. Sound has a unique ability to bypass the conscious mind and directly impact the body's stress response system, promoting relaxation and reducing tension. This can be accomplished by listening to calming music, engaging in guided sound meditations, or receiving sound healing treatments from a trained practitioner.

<u>Techniques for relaxation:</u>

Relaxation techniques in sound therapy encompass a wide range of practices and tools aimed at inducing a state of deep relaxation in the mind and body.

These techniques frequently involve the use of specific sounds, frequencies, rhythms, or vibrations to promote relaxation and reduce stress, such as binaural beats, Tibetan singing bowls, or guided imagery combined with soothing music. By engaging in relaxation techniques, individuals can activate the body's natural

<u>Managing Anxiety and Tension:</u>

Sound therapy has been shown to have a profound effect on the nervous system, helping to regulate emotions, reduce anxiety levels, and promote a sense of well-being. Sound-based techniques and practices, such as deep breathing exercises accompanied by calming music, progressive muscle relaxation, and guided imagery, are used to manage anxiety and tension.

CHAPTER 5
HEALING WITH SOUND

Sound therapy, a holistic approach to wellness, taps into the profound impact sound vibrations can have on the human body and mind. Rooted in ancient wisdom and increasingly supported by modern science, this therapeutic modality encompasses various techniques aimed at promoting healing, relaxation, and transformation. At its core, sound therapy operates on the principle that sound waves interact with the body's energy systems, affecting physiological processes and psychology.

<u>Sound Therapy for Physical Health.</u>

Sound therapy is a promising way to address a variety of physical health concerns by using the vibrational properties of sound to stimulate the body's natural healing mechanisms.

One of the primary applications of sound therapy is pain management, where specific frequencies are thought to alleviate discomfort by interrupting pain signals and promoting the release of endorphins, the body's natural painkillers. Sound therapy has also shown potential in

Sound Therapy for Emotional and Mental Wellness

Sound therapy, in addition to its physical advantages, has the potential to improve emotional and mental well-being. It can help manage conditions like depression, mood disorders, trauma, and difficulties with focus and concentration. Sound therapy techniques can provide a soothing and nurturing environment, fostering feelings of relaxation, safety, and emotional release.

Managing Depression and Mood Disorders

Sound therapy is a non-invasive and complementary approach to managing depression and mood disorders, providing individuals with alternative tools for self-care and emotional regulation. Sound baths, chanting, and listening to specific musical compositions can access states of deep relaxation and inner calm, counteracting feelings of sadness, anxiety, or agitation.

The rhythmic patterns and frequencies utilized in sound therapy

Supporting Trauma Recovery

Sound therapy offers a gentle and holistic approach to trauma recovery, providing individuals with tools to regulate their nervous system and release stored trauma from the body. Techniques such as sound massage, guided visualization, and breathwork accompanied by sound can be safely used to address the complex interplay of physical sensations, emotions, and cognitive patterns associated with traumatic experiences.

<u>Improving focus and concentration.</u>

In our fast-paced modern world, maintaining focus and concentration amidst distractions and demands can be challenging. Sound therapy offers innovative strategies for enhancing cognitive function and mental clarity, providing individuals with tools to optimize their attention and productivity. Certain sound frequencies and rhythms have been found to stimulate brainwave patterns associated with heightened focus and concentration, facilitating improved cognitive performance and task efficiency. Techniques such as binaural beats, which involve presenting slightly different frequencies to each ear, can induce a state of neural synchronization, enhancing cognitive processing and information retention. Moreover, sound therapy practices such as sound meditation and deep listening cultivate mindfulness and attentional control, allowing individuals to train their minds to stay present and focused amidst external stimuli.

By incorporating sound therapy into daily routines, individuals can cultivate a greater sense of mental clarity, resilience, and effectiveness in navigating life's challenges and opportunities.

sound therapy is a multifaceted approach to wellness that addresses the interconnected dimensions of physical health, emotional well-being, and mental clarity. By harnessing the power of sound vibrations, individuals can access profound states of relaxation, healing, and transformation, supporting their journey towards holistic wellness and vitality. As ancient wisdom converges with modern science, sound therapy continues to evolve

CHAPTER 6
SOUND THERAPY FOR SPECIFIC CONDITIONS

Sound therapy, also known as sound healing or sound meditation, has gained increasing recognition as a holistic approach to wellness that incorporates both ancient wisdom and modern scientific understanding. It employs the power of sound vibrations to promote healing, relaxation, and transformation at various levels of the human experience. In this comprehensive guide, we delve into the application of sound therapy for specific conditions, including chronic illnesses.

Chronic illnesses such as fibromyalgia, arthritis, and cancer present complex and debilitating symptoms that can significantly affect an individual's quality of life.

Sound therapy offers a non-invasive and complementary approach to conventional treatments, focusing on alleviating pain, reducing inflammation, and enhancing overall well-being. Fibromyalgia, characterized by widespread musculoskeletal pain and fatigue, may be alleviated through sound therapy techniques such as binaural beats and frequency-specific music, which can modulate brainwave activity and promote relaxation. Similarly, arthritis, a condition involving joint inflammation and stiffness, may benefit from sound therapy's ability to improve circulation, reduce muscle tension, and enhance mobility through resonant frequencies and vibrational therapies. Moreover, sound therapy has shown promise in supporting individuals undergoing cancer treatment, helping to manage pain, stress, and anxiety, and promoting emotional resilience and coping mechanisms through music therapy interventions and guided imagery techniques.

Neurological disorders encompass a broad spectrum of conditions affecting the brain and nervous system, posing significant challenges to cognitive, motor, and social functioning. Sound therapy offers a multidimensional approach to addressing these complex disorders, drawing upon principles of neuroplasticity, sensory integration, and emotional regulation. Alzheimer's disease, characterized by progressive cognitive decline and memory impairment, may benefit from sound therapy's potential to stimulate neural pathways, evoke memories, and enhance emotional connections through personalized playlists, familiar music, and rhythmic stimulation. Similarly, Parkinson's disease, a neurodegenerative disorder affecting movement and coordination, may be managed through rhythmic auditory stimulation techniques, which can improve gait, balance, and motor control by synchronizing movement with external auditory cues. Furthermore, autism spectrum disorders, characterized by social communication challenges and sensory sensitivities, may benefit from sound therapy interventions that promote sensory integration, emotional regulation, and social engagement through music-based interventions, sound baths, and therapeutic listening protocols tailored to individual needs.

sound therapy offers a holistic and integrative approach to managing chronic illnesses and neurological disorders, bridging ancient wisdom with modern science to promote healing, relaxation, and transformation.

By harnessing the power of sound vibrations and music therapy techniques, individuals can access a rich array of therapeutic benefits for physical, emotional, and cognitive well-being. As research in this field continues to evolve, sound therapy will

CHAPTER 7
ETHICS AND PROFESSIONAL PRACTICE.

Ethics and Professional Practice in Sound Therapy encompass a range of considerations vital for practitioners to uphold the integrity and effectiveness of their practice. Central to ethical practice is the recognition of the profound impact sound therapy can have on individuals' physical, emotional, and spiritual well-being. As a result, practitioners must adhere to strict ethical guidelines to ensure their clients' safety, confidentiality, and respect.

Ethical considerations in sound therapy include acknowledging the inherent power dynamics present in the therapeutic relationship.

Practitioners must maintain a commitment to beneficence and non-maleficence, ensuring that their interventions aim to promote healing and well-being while minimizing harm. This necessitates a thorough understanding of the potential risks and benefits of sound-based interventions and a willingness to prioritize the welfare of the client.

Client confidentiality and boundaries are fundamental principles that govern the therapeutic relationship in sound therapy. Practitioners must maintain strict confidentiality regarding their clients' personal information and treatment progress, ensuring that sensitive data is protected from unauthorized disclosure. Additionally, maintaining clear and consistent boundaries is essential to foster trust and safety within the therapeutic setting, establishing parameters for

Sound therapy practitioners must approach their work with humility and openness, actively recognizing and addressing the cultural implications of sound-based interventions, such as the use of specific instruments, techniques, or rituals that may hold significance in specific cultural contexts. Cultural sensitivity is essential in sound therapy to ensure that practitioners respect and honor their clients' diverse beliefs, values, and traditions.

Practitioners of sound therapy can improve the quality and consistency of their work by adhering to recognized standards of practice established by reputable professional organizations and undergoing rigorous training and certification processes.

Formal training programs should cover a wide range of topics, including the principles of sound healing, therapeutic techniques, anatomy and physiology, and ethical guidelines. Accreditation from reputable organizations serves as a mark of credibility and By adhering to a code of conduct, practitioners demonstrate their commitment to upholding ethical standards and promoting the welfare of their clients. A code of conduct serves as a guiding framework for ethical practice in sound therapy, outlining the principles, values, and behaviors expected of practitioners. It typically addresses issues such as professional integrity, respect for client autonomy, informed consent, and the appropriate use of therapeutic techniques.

CHAPTER 8
CASE STUDIES AND SUCCESS STORIES

Case studies and success stories in the realm of sound therapy provide invaluable insights into the efficacy and potential of this therapeutic modality. Through the detailed examination of individual cases, practitioners and researchers can discern patterns, outcomes, and best practices, thereby enhancing the understanding and application of sound therapy techniques. These studies typically involve the documentation and analysis of specific interventions using sound, such as sound baths, vibrational healing, or frequency-based treatments, and their impact on various aspects of health and well-being. By presenting concrete examples of how sound therapy has been utilized to address diverse conditions ranging from stress and anxiety to chronic pain and trauma, case studies offer compelling evidence of its effectiveness and versatility. Moreover, success stories highlight the transformative potential of sound therapy, illustrating how individuals have experienced profound healing, relaxation, and personal growth through their engagement with sound-based interventions. Through the dissemination of such narratives, practitioners and advocates can foster greater awareness and acceptance of sound therapy within both professional and lay communities, thereby facilitating its integration into mainstream healthcare practices.

Real-World Applications Of Sound Therapy

Real-life applications of sound therapy encompass a broad spectrum of contexts, ranging from clinical settings to holistic wellness practices and artistic expression.

In clinical settings, sound therapy techniques are increasingly being incorporated into conventional healthcare modalities, such as psychotherapy, physical rehabilitation, and pain management, to complement existing treatment protocols and enhance patient outcomes. For example, sound-based interventions like binaural beats or guided imagery with sound are being utilized alongside traditional psychotherapeutic approaches to alleviate symptoms of anxiety, depression, and post-traumatic stress disorder (PTSD). Similarly, in the field of physical rehabilitation, sound therapy modalities such as vibroacoustic therapy and rhythmic auditory stimulation have shown promise in improving motor function, gait dynamics, and overall mobility in individuals with neurological conditions like stroke or Parkinson's disease. Beyond clinical applications, sound therapy finds resonance in various wellness practices, including meditation, yoga, and mindfulness, where sound is employed as a tool for inducing relaxation, deepening introspection, and promoting spiritual connection. Moreover, the creative potential of sound therapy is manifested through avenues such as music therapy, sound healing concerts, and sound art installations, where sonic vibrations are harnessed for therapeutic, expressive, and aesthetic purposes. By elucidating the diverse applications of sound therapy across different domains of human experience, real-life examples underscore its versatility, accessibility, and relevance in contemporary society.

Case Studies Of Practitioners

Case studies from practitioners offer firsthand accounts of the application of sound therapy techniques in clinical or therapeutic settings, providing valuable insights into methodology, challenges, and outcomes. These studies typically document the experiences of practitioners as they work with clients or patients using various sound-based interventions, such as sound baths, tuning fork therapy, or voice analysis, to address specific health concerns or wellness goals. By detailing the process of assessment, intervention, and follow-up, practitioners elucidate the nuances of their approach, including the selection of appropriate sound tools, the design of personalized treatment protocols, and the integration of sound therapy within broader therapeutic frameworks.

 Moreover, case studies from practitioners often highlight the importance of the therapeutic relationship, empathic atonement, and client-centered care in optimizing the effectiveness of sound-based interventions. Through reflective analysis and clinical observations, practitioners glean valuable insights into the mechanisms of action underlying sound therapy modalities, as well as the factors influencing individual responses and outcomes. Furthermore, practitioner case studies serve as a platform for sharing best practices, innovative techniques, and lessons learned, thereby enriching the collective knowledge base of the sound therapy community and advancing the professionalization of the field.

Customer Testimonials

Testimonials from clients provide subjective accounts of the lived experiences and perceived benefits of sound therapy, offering poignant narratives that resonate with authenticity and emotional resonance.

As individuals share their personal journeys of healing, transformation, and self-discovery through sound-based interventions, their testimonials serve as powerful testimonials to the profound impact of sound on physical, emotional, and spiritual well-being.

Clients often describe how sound therapy has helped them alleviate symptoms of stress, anxiety, or chronic pain, enhance relaxation and sleep quality, and foster a greater sense of inner harmony and resilience.

Moreover, testimonials frequently highlight the holistic nature of the healing process, acknowledging the interconnectedness of mind, body, and spirit in the therapeutic journey.

By sharing their stories of hope, empowerment, and renewal, clients not only bear witness to the efficacy of sound therapy but also inspire others who may be seeking alternative paths to wellness and self-care. Furthermore, testimonials from clients contribute to the destigmatization and demystification of sound therapy, by normalizing its use and affirming its value within mainstream discourse on health and wellness.

As such, client testimonials play a vital role in raising awareness, generating interest, and building trust in the efficacy and accessibility of sound therapy as a viable therapeutic option for holistic well-being.

CONCLUSION

sound therapy represents a multifaceted approach to healing and transformation that integrates ancient wisdom, modern science, and practical techniques to promote holistic well-being. Through the targeted application of sound vibrations, frequencies, and rhythms, sound therapy modulates physiological, psychological, and energetic states, thereby eliciting a range of therapeutic effects, including relaxation, stress reduction, pain relief, and emotional release. Drawing on principles from disciplines such as music therapy, psychoacoustics, and energy medicine, sound therapy offers a diverse array of modalities and interventions tailored to individual needs and preferences. Case studies and success stories provide compelling evidence of the efficacy and versatility of sound therapy in addressing a wide range of health concerns and wellness goals, while testimonials from clients offer poignant narratives of personal transformation and empowerment. Moreover, practitioner case studies elucidate the intricacies of sound therapy practice, from assessment and intervention to therapeutic rapport and professional development.

As sound therapy continues to gain recognition and acceptance within mainstream healthcare and wellness settings, it holds promise as a valuable adjunctive modality for promoting holistic well-being and facilitating the journey towards wholeness and self-realization. By embracing the ancient wisdom of sound and harnessing the power of sound vibrations for healing, relaxation, and transformation, sound therapy offers a harmonious synthesis of art and science, spirit and matter, sound and silence, inviting individuals to tune into the symphony of their own inner resonance and reclaim their innate capacity for health, vitality, and joy.